THE DASH

COOKBOOK

The Guide to Lower your Blood Pressure
for Healthy Living.

Quick, Easy and Tasty Recipes with
Delicious Meals.

Low Sodium Dishes.

Alexangel Kitchen

Just for Our Readers

To Thank You for Purchasing the Book, for a limited time, you can get a Special FREE BOOK from Alexangel Kitchen

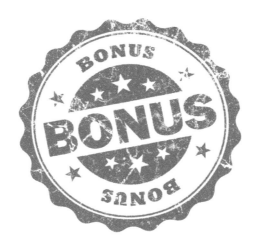

Just go to
https://alexangelkitchen.com/ to download your FREE BOOK

Table of Contents

The information in the following pages is broadly considered a truthful and accurate account of facts and as such, any inattention, use, or misuse of the information in question by the reader will render any resulting actions solely under their purview. There are no scenarios in which the publisher or the original author of this work can be in any fashion deemed liable for any hardship or damages that may befall them after undertaking information described herein.

Additionally, the information in the following pages is intended only for informational purposes and should thus be thought of as universal. As befitting its nature, it is presented without assurance regarding its prolonged validity or interim quality. Trademarks that are mentioned are done without written consent and can in no way be considered an endorsement from the trademark holder.

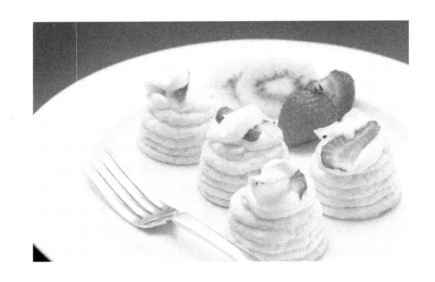

Side Dishes

Radish and Olives Salad

Preparation time: 5 minutes

Cooking time: 0 minutes

Servings: 4

Ingredients:

- 2 green onions, sliced

- 1-pound radishes, cubed

- 2 tablespoons balsamic vinegar

- 2 tablespoon olive oil

- 1 teaspoon chili powder

- 1 cup black olives, pitted and halved

- A pinch of black pepper

Directions:

1. Mix radishes with the onions and the other ingredients in a large salad bowl, toss, and serve as a side dish.

Nutrition:

Calories 123

Protein 1.3g

Carbohydrates 6.9g

Fat 10.8g

Fiber 3.3g

Sodium 345mg

Potassium 306mg

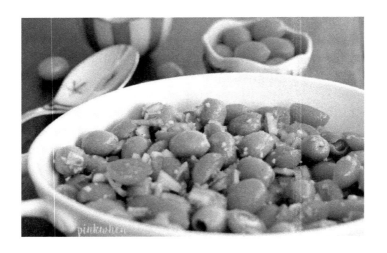

Spinach and Endives Salad

Preparation time: 5 minutes

Cooking time: 0 minutes

Servings: 4

Ingredients:

- 2 endives, roughly shredded

- 1 tablespoon dill, chopped

- ¼ cup lemon juice

- ¼ cup olive oil

- 2 cups baby spinach

- 2 tomatoes, cubed

- 1 cucumber, sliced

- ½ cups walnuts, chopped

Directions:

1. In a large bowl, combine the endives with the spinach and the other ingredients, toss and serve as a side dish.

Nutrition:

Calories 238

Protein 5.7g

Carbohydrates 8.4g

Fat 22.3g

Fiber 3.1g

Sodium 24mg

Potassium 506mg

Basil Olives Mix

Preparation time: 5 minutes
Cooking time: 0 minutes
Servings: 4
Ingredients:

- 2 tablespoons olive oil

- 1 tablespoon balsamic vinegar

- A pinch of black pepper

- 4 cups corn

- 2 cups black olives, pitted and halved

- 1 red onion, chopped

- ½ cup cherry tomatoes halved

- 1 tablespoon basil, chopped

- 1 tablespoon jalapeno, chopped

- 2 cups romaine lettuce, shredded

Directions:

1. Mix the corn with the olives, lettuce, and the other ingredients in a large bowl, toss well, divide between plates and serve as a side dish.

Nutrition:
Calories 290

Protein 6.2g

Carbohydrates 37.6g

Fat 16.1g

Fiber 7.4g

Sodium 613mg

Potassium 562mg

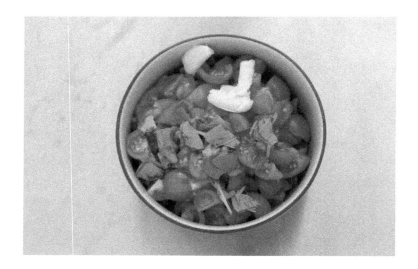

Arugula Salad

Preparation time: 5 minutes

Cooking time: 0 minutes

Servings: 4

Ingredients:

- ¼ cup pomegranate seeds

- 5 cups baby arugula

- 6 tablespoons green onions, chopped

- 1 tablespoon balsamic vinegar

- 2 tablespoons olive oil

- 3 tablespoons pine nuts

- ½ shallot, chopped

Directions:

1. In a salad bowl, combine the arugula with the pomegranate and the other ingredients, toss and serve.

Nutrition:

Calories 120

Protein 1.8g

Carbohydrates 4.2g

Fat 11.6g

Fiber 0.9g

Sodium 9mg

Potassium 163mg

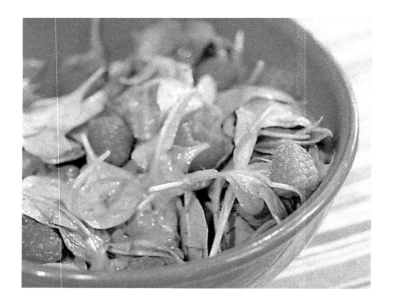

Spanish Rice

Preparation time: 15 minutes

Cooking time: 1 hour & 35 minutes

Servings: 8

Ingredients:

- Brown rice – 2 cups

- Extra virgin olive oil – .25 cup

- Garlic, minced – 2 cloves

- Onion, diced – 1

- Tomatoes, diced – 2

- Jalapeno, seeded and diced – 1

- Tomato paste – 1 tablespoon

- Cilantro, chopped - .5 cup

- Chicken broth, low-sodium – 2.5 cups

Directions:

1. Warm the oven to Fahrenheit 375 degrees. Puree the tomatoes, onion, plus garlic using a blender or food processor. Measure out two cups of this vegetable puree to use and discard the excess.

2. Into a large oven-safe Dutch pan, heat the extra virgin olive oil over medium heat until hot and

shimmering. Add in the jalapeno and rice to toast, cooking while occasionally stirring for two to three minutes.

3. Slowly stir the chicken broth into the rice, followed by the vegetable puree and tomato paste. Stir until combine and increase the heat to medium-high until the broth reaches a boil.

4. Cover the Dutch pan with an oven-safe lid, transfer the pot to the preheated oven, and bake within 1 hour and 15 minutes. Remove and stir the cilantro into the rice. Serve.

Nutrition:

Calories: 265

Sodium: 32mg

Potassium: 322mg

Carbs: 40g

Fat: 3g

Protein: 5g

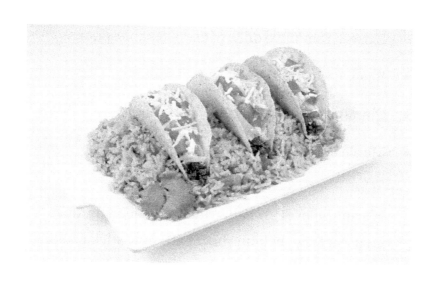

Sweet Potatoes and Apples

Preparation time: 15 minutes

Cooking time: 40 minutes

Servings: 4

Ingredients:

- Sweet potatoes, sliced into 1" cubes – 2

- Apples, cut into 1" cubes – 2

- Extra virgin olive oil, divided – 3 tablespoons

- Black pepper, ground - .25 teaspoon

- Cinnamon, ground – 1 teaspoon

- Maple syrup – 2 tablespoons

Directions:

1. Warm the oven to Fahrenheit 425 degrees and grease a large baking sheet with non-stick cooking spray. Toss the cubed sweet potatoes with two tablespoons of the olive oil and black pepper until coated. Roast the potatoes within twenty minutes, stirring them once halfway through the process.

2. Meanwhile, toss the apples with the remaining tablespoon of olive oil, cinnamon, and maple syrup until evenly coated. After the sweet potatoes have

cooked for twenty minutes, add the apples to the baking sheet and toss the sweet potatoes and apples.

3. Return to the oven, then roast it for twenty more minutes, once again giving it a good stir halfway through. Once the potatoes and apples are caramelized from the maple syrup, remove them from the oven and serve hot.

Nutrition:

Calories: 100

Carbs: 22g

Fat: 0g

Protein: 2g

Sodium: 38mg

Potassium: 341mg

Roasted Turnips

Preparation time: 15 minutes

Cooking time: 30 minutes

Servings: 4

Ingredients:

- Turnips, peels, and cut into ½" cubes – 2 cups

- Black pepper, ground - .25 teaspoon

- Garlic powder - .5 teaspoon

- Onion powder - .5 teaspoon

- Extra virgin olive oil – 1 tablespoon

Directions:

1. Warm the oven to Fahrenheit 400 degrees and prepare a large baking sheet, setting it aside. Begin by trimming the top and bottom edges off of the turnips and peeling them if you wish. Slice them into 1/2-inch cubes.

2. Toss the turnips with the extra virgin olive oil and seasonings and then spread them out on the prepared baking sheet. Roast the turnips until tender, stirring them halfway through, about thirty minutes in total.

Nutrition:

Calories: 50

Carbs: 5g

Fat: 4g

Protein: 1g

Sodium: 44mg

Potassium: 134mg

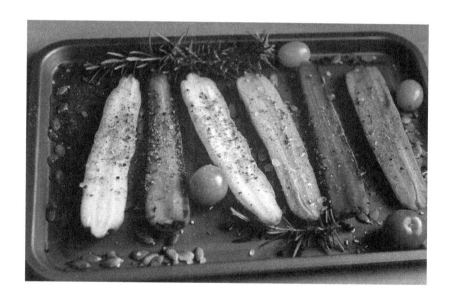

No-Mayo Potato Salad

Preparation time: 15 minutes

Cooking time: 20 minutes

Servings: 8

Ingredients:

- Red potatoes – 3 pounds

- Extra virgin olive oil - .5 cup

- White wine vinegar, divided – 5 tablespoons

- Dijon mustard – 2 teaspoons

- Red onion, sliced – 1 cup

- Black pepper, ground - .5 teaspoon

- Basil, fresh, chopped – 2 tablespoons

- Dill weed, fresh, chopped – 2 tablespoons

- Parsley, fresh, chopped – 2 tablespoons

Directions:

1. Add the red potatoes to a large pot and cover them with water until the water level is two inches above the potatoes. Put the pot on high heat, then boil potatoes until they are tender when poked with a fork, about fifteen to twenty minutes. Drain off the water.

2. Let the potatoes to cool until they can easily be handled but are still warm, then cut it in half and put them in a large bowl. Stir in three tablespoons of the white wine vinegar, giving the potatoes a good stir so that they can evenly absorb the vinegar.

3. Mix the rest of two tablespoons of vinegar, extra virgin olive oil, Dijon mustard, and black pepper in a small bowl. Add this mixture to the potatoes and give them a good toss to thoroughly coat the potatoes.

4. Toss in the red onion and minced herbs. Serve at room temperature or chilled. Serve immediately or store in the fridge for up to four days.

Nutrition:

Calories: 144

Carbs: 19g

Fat: 7g

Protein: 2g

Sodium: 46mg

Potassium: 814mg

Zucchini Tomato Bake

Preparation time: 15 minutes

Cooking time: 30 minutes

Servings: 4

Ingredients:

- Grape tomatoes, cut in half – 10 ounces

- Zucchini – 2

- Garlic, minced – 5 cloves

- Italian herb seasoning – 1 teaspoon

- Black pepper, ground - .25 teaspoon

- Parsley, fresh, chopped - .33 cup

- Parmesan cheese, low-sodium, grated - .5 cup

Directions:

1. Warm the oven to Fahrenheit 350 degrees and coat a large baking sheet with non-stick cooking spray. Mix the tomatoes, zucchini, garlic, Italian herb seasoning, Black pepper, and Parmesan cheese in a bowl.

2. Put the mixture out on the baking sheet and roast until the zucchini for thirty minutes. Remove, and garnish with parsley over the top before serving.

Nutrition:

Calories: 35

Carbs: 4g

Fat: 2g

Protein: 2g

Sodium: 30mg

Potassium: 649mg

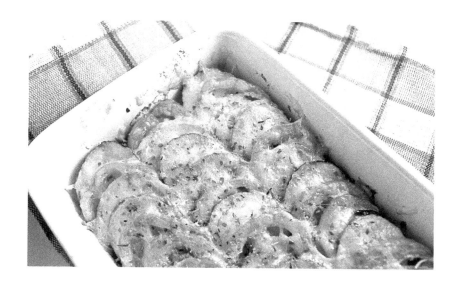

Creamy Broccoli Cheddar Rice

Preparation time: 15 minutes

Cooking time: 40 minutes

Servings: 6

Ingredients:

- Brown rice – 1 cup

- Chicken broth, low-sodium – 2 cups

- Onion, minced – 1

- Extra virgin olive oil, divided – 3 tablespoons

- Garlic, minced – 2 cloves

- Skim milk - .5 cup

- Black pepper, ground - .25 teaspoon

- Broccoli, chopped – 1.5 cups

- Cheddar cheese, low-sodium, shredded – 1 cup

Directions:

1. Put one tablespoon of the extra virgin olive oil in a large pot and sauté the onion plus garlic over medium heat within two minutes.

2. Put the chicken broth in a pot and wait for it to come to a boil before adding in the rice. Simmer the rice over low heat for twenty-five minutes.

3. Stir the skim milk, black pepper, and remaining two tablespoons of olive oil into the rice. Simmer again within five more minutes. Stir in the broccoli and cook the rice for five more minutes, until the broccoli is tender. Stir in the rice and serve while warm.

Nutrition:

Calories: 200

Carbs: 33g

Fat: 3g

Protein: 10g

Sodium: 50mg

Potassium: 344mg

Smashed Brussels Sprouts

Preparation time: 15 minutes

Cooking time: 40 minutes

Servings: 6

Ingredients:

- Brussels sprouts – 2 pounds

- Garlic, minced – 3 cloves

- Balsamic vinegar – 3 tablespoons

- Extra virgin olive oil - .5 cup

- Black pepper, ground - .5 teaspoon

- Leek washed and thinly sliced – 1

- Parmesan cheese, low-sodium, grated - .5 cup

Directions:

1. Warm the oven to Fahrenheit 450 degrees and prepare two large baking sheets. Trim the yellow leaves and stems off of the Brussels sprouts and then steam them until tender, about twenty to twenty-five minutes.

2. Mix the garlic, black pepper, balsamic vinegar, and extra virgin olive oil in a large bowl. Add the steamed Brussels sprouts and leeks to the bowl and toss until evenly coated.

3. Spread the Brussels sprouts and leaks divided onto the prepared baking sheets.

4. Use a fork or a glass and press down on each of the Brussels sprouts to create flat patties. Put the Parmesan cheese on top and place the smashed sprouts in the oven for fifteen minutes until crispy. Enjoy hot and fresh from the oven.

Nutrition:

Calories: 116

Carbs: 11g

Fat: 5g

Protein: 10g

Sodium: 49mg

Potassium: 642mg

Cilantro Lime Rice

Preparation time: 15 minutes

Cooking time: 40 minutes

Servings: 6

Ingredients:

- Brown rice – 1.5 cups

- Lime juice – 2 tablespoons

- Lemon juice – 1.5 teaspoons

- Lime zest - .5 teaspoon

- Cilantro, chopped - .25 cup

- Bay leaf – 1

- Extra virgin olive oil – 1 tablespoon

- Water

Directions:

1. Cook rice and bay leaf in a pot with boiling water. Mix the mixture and allow it to boil for thirty minutes, reducing the heat slightly if need be.

2. Once the rice is tender, drain off the water and return the rice to the pot. Let it sit off of the heat within ten minutes. Remove the bay leaf and use a

fork to fluff the rice. Stir the rest of the fixing into the rice and then serve immediately.

Nutrition:

Calories: 94

Carbs: 15g

Fat: 3g

Protein: 2g

Sodium: 184mg

Potassium: 245mg

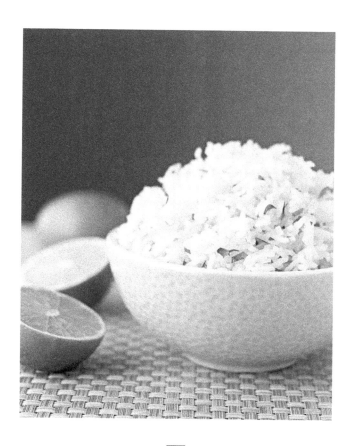

Corn Salad with Lime Vinaigrette

Preparation time: 15 minutes

Cooking time: 7 minutes

Servings: 6

Ingredients:

- Corn kernels, fresh – 4.5 cups

- Lemon juice – 1 tablespoon

- Red bell pepper, diced – 1

- Grape tomatoes halved – 1 cup

- Cilantro, chopped - .25 cup

- Green onion, chopped - .25 cup

- Jalapeno, diced – 1

- Red onion, thinly sliced - .25

- Feta cheese - .5 cup

- Truvia baking blend – 2 tablespoons

- Extra virgin olive oil – 2 tablespoons

- Honey - .5 tablespoon

- Lime juice – 3 tablespoons

- Black pepper, ground - .125 teaspoon

- Cayenne pepper, ground - .125 teaspoon

- Garlic powder - .125 teaspoon

- Onion powder - .125 teaspoon

Directions:

1. To create your lime vinaigrette, add the lime juice, onion powder, garlic powder, black pepper, cayenne pepper, and honey to a bowl. Mix, then slowly add in the extra virgin olive oil while whisking vigorously.

2. Boil a pot of water and add in the lemon juice, Baking Truvia, and corn kernels. Allow the corn to boil for seven minutes until tender. Strain the boiling water and add the corn kernels to a bowl of ice water to stop the cooking process and cool the kernels. Drain off the ice water and reserve the corn.

3. Add the tomatoes, red pepper, jalapeno, green onion, red onion, cilantro, and cooked corn to a large bowl and toss it until the vegetables are well distributed. Add the feta cheese and vinaigrette to the vegetables and then toss until well combined and evenly coated. Serve immediately.

Nutrition:
Calories: 88
Carbs: 23g
Fat: 0g

Protein: 3g

Sodium: 124mg

Potassium: 508mg

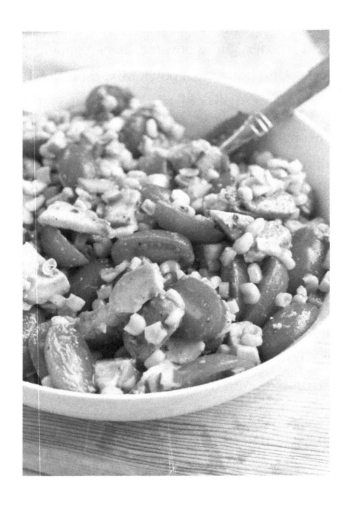

Mediterranean Chickpea Salad

Preparation time: 15 minutes

Cooking time: 0 minutes

Servings: 6

Ingredients:

- Chickpeas, cooked – 4 cups

- Bell pepper, diced – 2 cups

- Cucumber, chopped – 1 cup

- Tomato, chopped – 1 cup

- Avocado, diced – 1

- Red wine vinegar – 2.5 tablespoons

- Lemon juice – 1 tablespoon

- Extra virgin olive oil – 3 tablespoons

- Parsley, fresh, chopped – 1 teaspoon

- Oregano, dried - .5 teaspoon

- Garlic, minced – 1 teaspoon

- Dill weed, dried - .25 teaspoon

- Black pepper, ground - .25 teaspoon

Directions:

1. Add the diced vegetables except for the avocado and the chickpeas to a large bowl and toss them. In a separate bowl, whisk the seasonings, lemon juice, red wine vinegar, and extra virgin olive oil to create a vinaigrette. Once combined, pour the mixture over the salad and toss to combine.

2. Place the salad in the fridge and allow it to marinate for at least a couple of hours before serving or up to two days. Immediately before serving the salad, dice the avocado and toss it in.

Nutrition:

Calories: 120

Carbs: 14g

Fat: 5g

Protein: 4g

Sodium: 15mg

Potassium: 696mg

Italian Roasted Cabbage

Preparation time: 15 minutes

Cooking time: 15 minutes

Servings: 8

Ingredients:

- Cabbage, sliced into 8 wedges – 1

- Black pepper, ground – 1.5 teaspoons

- Extra virgin olive oil - .66 cup

- Italian herb seasoning – 2 teaspoons

- Parmesan cheese, low-sodium, grated - .66 cup

Directions:

1. Warm the oven to Fahrenheit 425 degrees. Prepare a large lined baking sheet with aluminum foil and then spray it with non-stick cooking spray.

2. Slice your cabbage in half, remove the stem, and then cut each half into four wedges so that you are left with eight wedges in total.

3. Arrange the cabbage wedges on the baking sheet and then drizzle half of the extra virgin olive oil over them. Sprinkle half of the seasonings and Parmesan cheese over the top.

4. Place the baking sheet in the hot oven, allow the cabbage to roast for fifteen minutes, and then flip the wedges. Put the rest of the olive oil over the top and then sprinkle the remaining seasonings and cheese over the top as well.

5. Return the cabbage to the oven and allow it to roast for fifteen more minutes, until tender. Serve fresh and hot.

Nutrition:

Calories: 17

Carbs: 4g

Fat: 0g

Protein: 1g

Sodium: 27mg

Potassium: 213mg

Tex-Mex Cole Slaw

Preparation time: 15 minutes

Cooking time: 0 minutes

Servings: 12

Ingredients:

- Black beans, cooked – 2 cups

- Grape tomatoes, sliced in half – 1.5 cups

- Grilled corn kernels – 1.5 cups

- Jalapeno, seeded and minced – 1

- Cilantro, chopped – .5 cup

- Bell pepper, diced – 1

- Coleslaw cabbage mix – 16 ounces

- Lime juice – 3 tablespoons

- Light sour cream - .66 cup

- Olive oil mayonnaise, reduced-fat – 1 cup

- Chili powder – 1 tablespoon

- Cumin, ground – 1 teaspoon

- Onion powder – 1 teaspoon

- Garlic powder – 1 teaspoon

Directions:

1. Mix the sour cream, mayonnaise, lime juice, garlic powder, onion powder, cumin, and chili powder in a bowl to create the dressing.

2. In a large bowl, toss the vegetables and then add in the prepared dressing and toss again until evenly coated. Chill the mixture in the fridge for thirty minutes to twelve hours before serving.

Nutrition:

Calories: 50

Carbs: 10g

Fat: 1g

Protein: 3g

Sodium: 194mg

Potassium: 345mg

Roasted Okra

Preparation time: 15 minutes

Cooking time: 20 minutes

Servings: 4

Ingredients:

- Okra, fresh – 1 pound

- Extra virgin olive oil – 2 tablespoons

- Cayenne pepper, ground - .125 teaspoon

- Paprika – 1 teaspoon

- Garlic powder - .25 teaspoon

Directions:

1. Warm the oven to Fahrenheit 450 degrees and prepare a large baking sheet. Cut the okra into pieces appropriate 1/2-inch in size.

2. Place the okra on the baking pan and top it with the olive oil and seasonings, giving it a good toss until evenly coated. Roast the okra in the heated oven until it is tender and lightly browned and seared. Serve immediately while hot.

Nutrition:

Calories: 65

Carbs: 6g

Fat: 5g

Protein: 2g

Sodium: 9mg

Potassium: 356mg

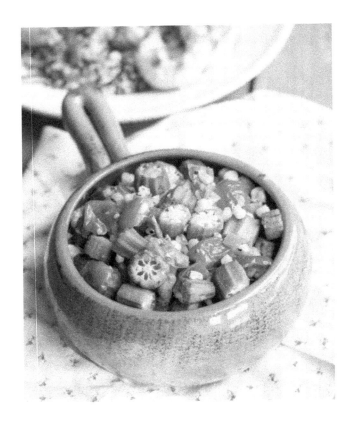

Brown Sugar Glazed Carrots

Preparation time: 15 minutes

Cooking time: 25 minutes

Servings: 6

Ingredients:

- Carrots, sliced into 1-inch pieces – 2 pounds

- Light olive oil - .33 cup

- Truvia Brown Sugar Blend - .25 cup

- Black pepper, ground - .25 teaspoon

Directions:

1. Warm the oven to Fahrenheit 400 degrees and prepare a large baking sheet. Toss the carrots with the oil, Truvia, and black pepper until evenly coated and then spread them out on the prepared baking sheet.

2. Place the carrots in the oven and allow them to roast until tender, about twenty to twenty-five minutes. Halfway through the cooking time, give the carrots a good serve. Remove the carrots from the oven and serve them alone or topped with fresh parsley.

Nutrition:

Calories: 110

Carbs: 16g

Fat: 4g

Protein: 1g

Sodium: 105mg

Potassium: 486mg

Oven-Roasted Beets with Honey Ricotta

Preparation time: 15 minutes

Cooking time: 40 minutes

Servings: 6

Ingredients:

- Purple beets – 1 pound

- Golden beets – 1 pound

- Ricotta cheese, low-fat - .5 cup

- Extra virgin olive oil – 3 tablespoons

- Honey – 1 tablespoon

- Rosemary, fresh, chopped – 1 teaspoon

- Black pepper, ground - .25 teaspoon

Directions:

1. Warm the oven to Fahrenheit 375 degrees and prepare a large baking sheet by lining it with kitchen parchment. Slice the beets into 1/2-inch cubes before tossing them with the extra virgin olive oil and black pepper.

2. Put the beets on the prepared baking sheet and allow them to roast until tender, about thirty-five to

forty minutes. Halfway through the cooking process, flip the beets over.

3. Meanwhile, in a small bowl, whisk the ricotta with the rosemary and honey. Fridge until ready to serve. Once the beets are done cooking, serve them topped with the ricotta mixture, and enjoy.

Nutrition:

Calories: 195

Carbs: 24g

Fat: 8g

Protein: 8g

Sodium: 139mg

Potassium: 521mg

Easy Carrots Mix

Preparation time: 10 minutes

Cooking time: 40 minutes

Servings: 6

Ingredients:

- 15 carrots, halved lengthwise

- 2 tablespoons coconut sugar

- ¼ cup olive oil

- ½ teaspoon rosemary, dried

- ½ teaspoon garlic powder

- A pinch of black pepper

Directions:

1. In a bowl, combine the carrots with the sugar, oil, rosemary, garlic powder, and black pepper, toss well, spread on a lined baking sheet, introduce in the oven and bake at 400 degrees F for 40 minutes. Serve.

Nutrition:

Calories: 60

Carbs: 9g

Fat: 0g

Protein: 2g

Sodium: 0 mg

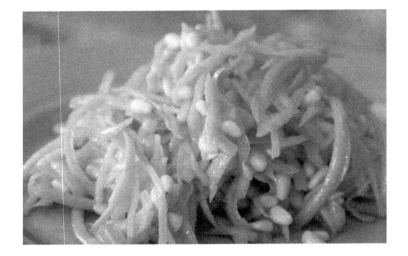

Tasty Grilled Asparagus

Preparation time: 10 minutes

Cooking time: 6 minutes

Servings: 4

Ingredients:

- 2 pounds asparagus, trimmed

- 2 tablespoons olive oil

- A pinch of salt and black pepper

Directions:

1. In a bowl, combine the asparagus with salt, pepper, and oil and toss well. Place the asparagus on a preheated grill over medium-high heat, cook for 3 minutes on each side, then serve.

Nutrition:

Calories: 50

Carbs: 8g

Fat: 1g

Protein: 5g

Sodium: 420 mg

Roasted Carrots

Preparation time: 10 minutes

Cooking time: 30 minutes

Servings: 4

Ingredients:

- 2 pounds carrots, quartered

- A pinch of black pepper

- 3 tablespoons olive oil

- 2 tablespoons parsley, chopped

Directions:

1. Arrange the carrots on a lined baking sheet, add black pepper and oil, toss, introduce in the oven, and cook within 30 minutes at 400 degrees F. Add parsley, toss, divide between plates and serve as a side dish.

Nutrition:

Calories: 89

Carbs: 10g

Fat: 6g

Protein: 1g

Sodium: 0 mg

Oven Roasted Asparagus

Preparation time: 10 minutes

Cooking time: 25 minutes

Servings: 4

Ingredients:

- 2 pounds asparagus spears, trimmed

- 3 tablespoons olive oil

- A pinch of black pepper

- 2 teaspoons sweet paprika

- 1 teaspoon sesame seeds

Directions:

1. Arrange the asparagus on a lined baking sheet, add oil, black pepper, and paprika, toss, introduce in the oven and bake within 25 minutes at 400 degrees F. Divide the asparagus between plates, sprinkle sesame seeds on top, and serve as a side dish.

Nutrition:

Calories: 45

Carbs: 5g

Fat: 2g

Protein: 2g

Sodium: 0 mg

Baked Potato with Thyme

Preparation time: 10 minutes

Cooking time: 1 hour and 15 minutes

Servings: 8

Ingredients:

- 6 potatoes, peeled and sliced

- 2 garlic cloves, minced

- 2 tablespoons olive oil

- 1 and ½ cups of coconut cream

- ¼ cup of coconut milk

- 1 tablespoon thyme, chopped

- ¼ teaspoon nutmeg, ground

- A pinch of red pepper flakes

- 1 and ½ cups low-fat cheddar, shredded

- ½ cup low-fat parmesan, grated

Directions:

1. Heat-up a pan with the oil over medium heat, add garlic, stir and cook for 1 minute. Add coconut cream, coconut milk, thyme, nutmeg, and pepper flakes, stir, bring to a simmer, adjust to low and cook within 10 minutes.

2. Put one-third of the potatoes in a baking dish, add 1/3 of the cream, repeat the process with the remaining potatoes and the cream, sprinkle the cheddar on top, cover with tin foil, introduce in the oven and cook at 375 degrees F for 45 minutes. Uncover the dish, sprinkle the parmesan, bake everything for 20 minutes, divide between plates, and serve as a side dish.

Nutrition:

Calories: 132

Carbs: 21g

Fat: 4g

Protein: 2g

Sodium: 56 mg

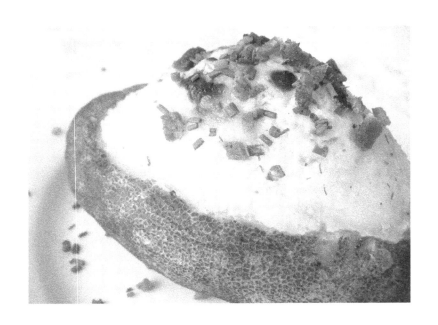

Spicy Brussels Sprouts

Preparation time: 10 minutes

Cooking time: 20 minutes

Servings: 6

Ingredients:

- 2 pounds Brussels sprouts, halved

- 2 tablespoons olive oil

- A pinch of black pepper

- 1 tablespoon sesame oil

- 2 garlic cloves, minced

- ½ cup coconut aminos

- 2 teaspoons apple cider vinegar

- 1 tablespoon coconut sugar

- 2 teaspoons chili sauce

- A pinch of red pepper flakes

- Sesame seeds for serving

Directions:

1. Spread the sprouts on a lined baking dish, add the olive oil, the sesame oil, black pepper, garlic, aminos, vinegar, coconut sugar, chili sauce, and pepper flakes, toss well, introduce in the oven and

bake within 20 minutes at 425 degrees F. Divide the sprouts between plates, sprinkle sesame seeds on top and serve as a side dish.

Nutrition:

Calories: 64

Carbs: 13g

Fat: 0g

Protein: 4g

Sodium: 314 mg

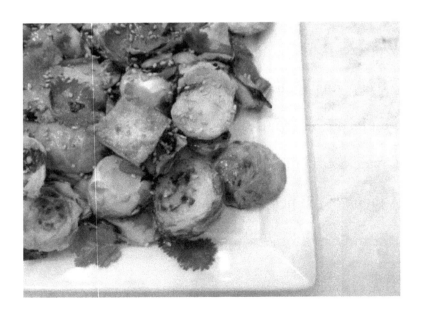

Baked Cauliflower with Chili

Preparation time: 10 minutes

Cooking time: 30 minutes

Servings: 4

Ingredients:

- 3 tablespoons olive oil

- 2 tablespoons chili sauce

- Juice of 1 lime

- 3 garlic cloves, minced

- 1 cauliflower head, florets separated

- A pinch of black pepper

- 1 teaspoon cilantro, chopped

Directions:

1. In a bowl, combine the oil with the chili sauce, lime juice, garlic, and black pepper and whisk. Add cauliflower florets, toss, spread on a lined baking sheet, introduce in the oven and bake at 425 degrees F for 30 minutes. Divide the cauliflower between plates, sprinkle cilantro on top, and serve as a side dish.

Nutrition:

Calories: 31

Carbs: 3g

Fat: 0g

Protein: 3g

Sodium: 4 mg

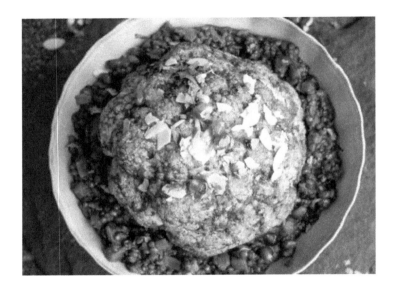

Baked Broccoli

Preparation time: 10 minutes

Cooking time: 15 minutes

Servings: 4

Ingredients:

- 1 tablespoon olive oil

- 1 broccoli head, florets separated

- 2 garlic cloves, minced

- ½ cup coconut cream

- ½ cup low-fat mozzarella, shredded

- ¼ cup low-fat parmesan, grated

- A pinch of pepper flakes, crushed

Directions:

1. In a baking dish, combine the broccoli with oil, garlic, cream, pepper flakes, mozzarella, and toss. Sprinkle the parmesan on top, introduce in the oven and bake at 375 degrees F for 15 minutes. Serve.

Nutrition:

Calories: 90

Carbs: 6g

Fat: 7g

Protein: 3g

Sodium: 30 mg

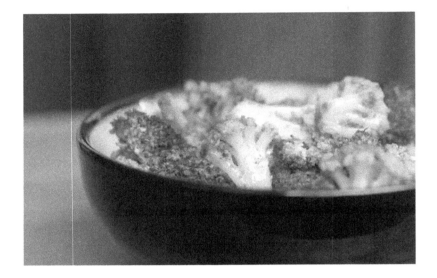

Slow Cooked Potatoes with Cheddar

Preparation time: 10 minutes

Cooking time: 6 hours

Servings: 6

Ingredients:

- Cooking spray

- 2 pounds baby potatoes, quartered

- 3 cups low-fat cheddar cheese, shredded

- 2 garlic cloves, minced

- 8 bacon slices, cooked and chopped

- ¼ cup green onions, chopped

- 1 tablespoon sweet paprika

- A pinch of black pepper

Directions:

1. Spray a slow cooker with the cooking spray, add baby potatoes, cheddar, garlic, bacon, green onions, paprika, and black pepper, toss, cover, and cook on High for 6 hours. Serve.

Nutrition:

Calories: 112

Carbs: 26g

Fat: 4g

Protein: 8g

Sodium: 234 mg

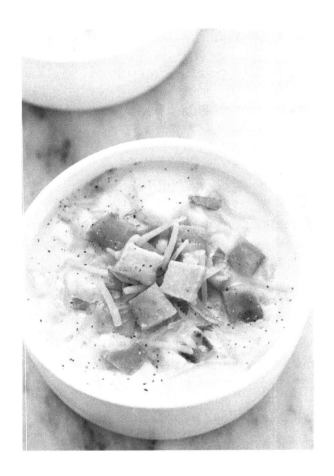

Squash Salad with Orange

Preparation time: 10 minutes

Cooking time: 30 minutes

Servings: 6

Ingredients:

- 1 cup of orange juice

- 3 tablespoons coconut sugar

- 1 and ½ tablespoons mustard

- 1 tablespoon ginger, grated

- 1 and ½ pounds butternut squash, peeled and roughly cubed

- Cooking spray

- A pinch of black pepper

- 1/3 cup olive oil

- 6 cups salad greens

- 1 radicchio, sliced

- ½ cup pistachios, roasted

Directions:

1. Mix the orange juice with the sugar, mustard, ginger, black pepper, squash in a bowl, toss well, spread on a lined baking sheet, spray everything

with cooking oil, and bake for 30 minutes 400 degrees F.

2. In a salad bowl, combine the squash with salad greens, radicchio, pistachios, and oil, toss well, then serve.

Nutrition:

Calories: 17

Carbs: 2g

Fat: 0g

Protein: 0g

Sodium: 0 mg

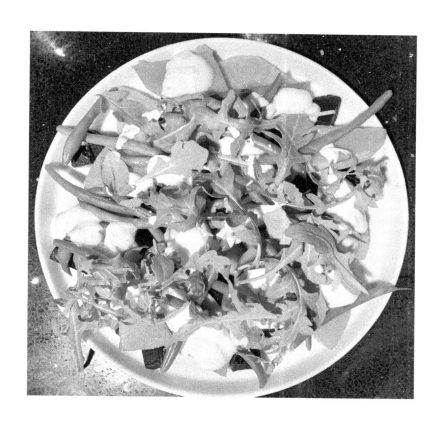

Colored Iceberg Salad

Preparation time: 10 minutes

Cooking time: 0 minutes

Servings: 4

Ingredients:

- 1 iceberg lettuce head, leaves torn

- 6 bacon slices, cooked and halved

- 2 green onions, sliced

- 3 carrots, shredded

- 6 radishes, sliced

- ¼ cup red vinegar

- ¼ cup olive oil

- 3 garlic cloves, minced

- A pinch of black pepper

Directions:

1. Mix the lettuce leaves with the bacon, green onions, carrots, radishes, vinegar, oil, garlic, and black pepper in a large salad bowl, toss, divide between plates and serve as a side dish.

Nutrition:

Calories: 15

Carbs: 3g

Fat: 0g

Protein: 1g

Sodium: 15 mg

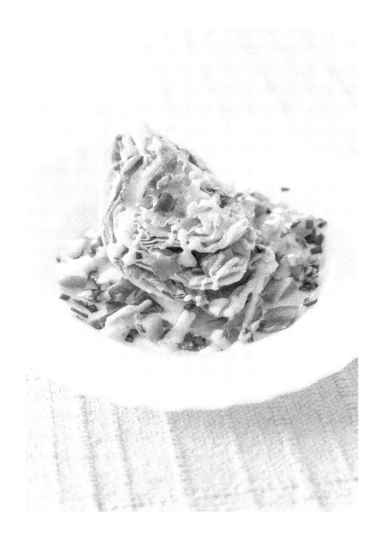

Fennel Salad with Arugula

Preparation time: 10 minutes

Cooking time: 0 minutes

Servings: 4

Ingredients:

- 2 fennel bulbs, trimmed and shaved

- 1 and ¼ cups zucchini, sliced

- 2/3 cup dill, chopped

- ¼ cup lemon juice

- ¼ cup olive oil

- 6 cups arugula

- ½ cups walnuts, chopped

- 1/3 cup low-fat feta cheese, crumbled

Directions:

1. Mix the fennel with the zucchini, dill, lemon juice, arugula, oil, walnuts, and cheese in a large bowl, toss, then serve.

Nutrition:

Calories: 65

Carbs: 6g

Fat: 5g

Protein: 1g

Sodium: 140 mg

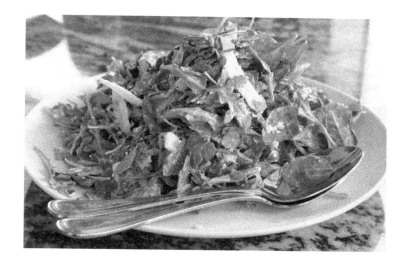

Corn Mix

Preparation time: 10 minutes

Cooking time: 0 minutes

Servings: 4

Ingredients:

- ½ cup cider vinegar

- ¼ cup of coconut sugar

- A pinch of black pepper

- 4 cups corn

- ½ cup red onion, chopped

- ½ cup cucumber, sliced

- ½ cup red bell pepper, chopped

- ½ cup cherry tomatoes halved

- 3 tablespoons parsley, chopped

- 1 tablespoon basil, chopped

- 1 tablespoon jalapeno, chopped

- 2 cups baby arugula leaves

Directions:

1. Mix the corn with onion, cucumber, bell pepper, cherry tomatoes, parsley, basil, jalapeno, and

arugula in a large bowl. Add vinegar, sugar, and black pepper, toss well, divide between plates and serve as a side dish.

Nutrition:
Calories: 110
Carbs: 25g
Fat: 0g
Protein: 2g
Sodium: 120 mg

Persimmon Salad

Preparation time: 10 minutes

Cooking time: 0 minutes

Servings: 4

Ingredients:

- Seeds from 1 pomegranate

- 2 persimmons, cored and sliced

- 5 cups baby arugula

- 6 tablespoons green onions, chopped

- 4 navel oranges, cut into segments

- ¼ cup white vinegar

- 1/3 cup olive oil

- 3 tablespoons pine nuts

- 1 and ½ teaspoons orange zest, grated

- 2 tablespoons orange juice

- 1 tablespoon coconut sugar

- ½ shallot, chopped

- A pinch of cinnamon powder

Directions:

1. In a salad bowl, combine the pomegranate seeds with persimmons, arugula, green onions, and oranges and toss. In another bowl, combine the vinegar with the oil, pine nuts, orange zest, orange juice, sugar, shallot, and cinnamon, whisk well, add to the salad, toss and serve as a side dish.

Nutrition:

Calories: 310

Carbs: 33g

Fat: 16g

Protein: 7g

Sodium: 320 mg

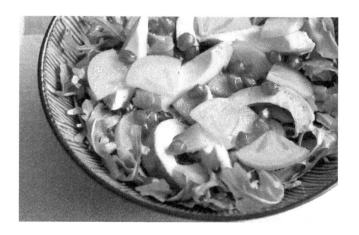

Avocado Side Salad

Preparation time: 10 minutes

Cooking time: 0 minutes

Servings: 4

Ingredients:

- 4 blood oranges, slice into segments

- 2 tablespoons olive oil

- A pinch of red pepper, crushed

- 2 avocados, peeled, cut into wedges

- 1 and ½ cups baby arugula

- ¼ cup almonds, toasted and chopped

- 1 tablespoon lemon juice

Directions:

1. Mix the oranges with the oil, red pepper, avocados, arugula, almonds, and lemon juice in a bowl, then serve.

Nutrition:

Calories: 146

Carbs: 8g

Fat: 7g

Protein: 15g

Sodium: 320 mg

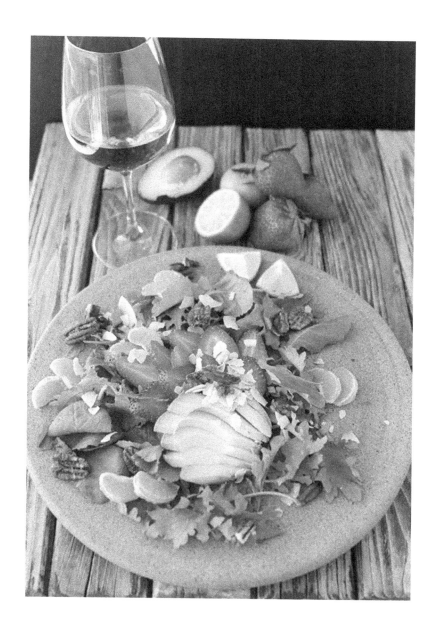

Spiced Broccoli Florets

Preparation time: 10 minutes

Cooking time: 3 hours

Servings: 10

Ingredients:

- 6 cups broccoli florets

- 1 and ½ cups low-fat cheddar cheese, shredded

- ½ teaspoon cider vinegar

- ¼ cup yellow onion, chopped

- 10 ounces tomato sauce, sodium-free

- 2 tablespoons olive oil

- A pinch of black pepper

Directions:

1. Grease your slow cooker with the oil, add broccoli, tomato sauce, cider vinegar, onion, and black pepper, cook on High within 2 hours, and 30 minutes. Sprinkle the cheese all over, cover, cook on High for 30 minutes more, divide between plates, and serve as a side dish.

Nutrition:

Calories 119

Fat 8.7g

Sodium 272mg

Carbohydrate 5.7g

Fiber 1.9g

Sugars 2.3g

Protein 6.2g

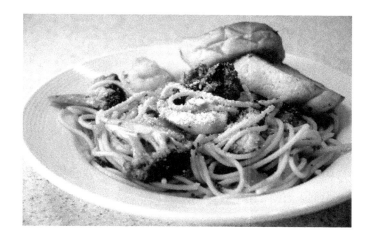

Lima Beans Dish

Preparation time: 10 minutes

Cooking time: 5 hours

Servings: 10

Ingredients:

- 1 green bell pepper, chopped

- 1 sweet red pepper, chopped

- 1 and ½ cups tomato sauce, salt-free

- 1 yellow onion, chopped

- ½ cup of water

- 16 ounces canned kidney beans, no-salt-added, drained and rinsed

- 16 ounces canned black-eyed peas, no-salt-added, drained and rinsed

- 15 ounces corn

- 15 ounces canned lima beans, no-salt-added, drained and rinsed

- 15 oz canned black beans, no-salt-added, drained

- 2 celery ribs, chopped

- 2 bay leaves

- 1 teaspoon ground mustard

- 1 tablespoon cider vinegar

Directions:

1. In your slow cooker, mix the tomato sauce with the onion, celery, red pepper, green bell pepper, water, bay leaves, mustard, vinegar, kidney beans, black-eyed peas, corn, lima beans, and black beans, cook on Low within 5 hours. Discard bay leaves, divide the whole mix between plates, and serve.

Nutrition:

Calories 602

Fat 4.8g

Sodium 255mg

Carbohydrate 117.7g

Fiber 24.6g

Sugars 13.4g

Protein 33g

Soy Sauce Green Beans

Preparation time: 10 minutes

Cooking time: 2 hours

Servings: 12

Ingredients:

- 3 tablespoons olive oil

- 16 ounces green beans

- ½ teaspoon garlic powder

- ½ cup of coconut sugar

- 1 teaspoon low-sodium soy sauce

Directions:

1. In your slow cooker, mix the green beans with the oil, sugar, soy sauce, and garlic powder, cover, and cook on Low for 2 hours. Toss the beans, divide them between plates, and serve as a side dish.

Nutrition:

Calories 46

Fat 3.6g

Sodium 29mg

Carbohydrate 3.6g

Fiber 1.3g

Sugars 0.6g

Protein 0.8g

Butter Corn

Preparation time: 10 minutes

Cooking time: 4 hours

Servings: 12

Ingredients:

- 20 ounces fat-free cream cheese

- 10 cups corn

- ½ cup low-fat butter

- ½ cup fat-free milk

- A pinch of black pepper

- 2 tablespoons green onions, chopped

Directions:

1. In your slow cooker, mix the corn with cream cheese, milk, butter, black pepper, and onions, cook on Low within 4 hours. Toss one more time, divide between plates and serve as a side dish.

Nutrition:

Calories 279

Fat 18g

Cholesterol 52mg

Sodium 165mg

Carbohydrate 26g

Fiber 3.5g

Sugars 4.8g

Protein 8.1g

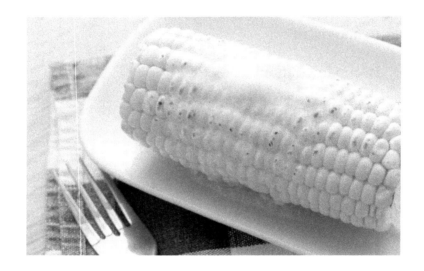

Stevia Peas with Marjoram

Preparation time: 10 minutes

Cooking time: 5 hours

Servings: 12

Ingredients:

- 1-pound carrots, sliced

- 1 yellow onion, chopped

- 16 ounces peas

- 2 tablespoons stevia

- 2 tablespoons olive oil

- 4 garlic cloves, minced

- ¼ cup of water

- 1 teaspoon marjoram, dried

- A pinch of white pepper

Directions:

1. In your slow cooker, mix the carrots with water, onion, oil, stevia, garlic, marjoram, white pepper, peas, toss, cover, and cook on High for 5 hours. Divide between plates and serve as a side dish.

Nutrition:

Calories 71

Fat 2.5g

Sodium 29mg

Carbohydrate 12.1g

Fiber 3.1g

Sugars 4.4g

Protein 2.5g

Potassium 231mg

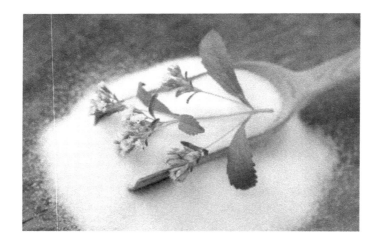

Pilaf with Bella Mushrooms

Preparation time: 10 minutes

Cooking time: 3 hours

Servings: 6

Ingredients:

- 1 cup wild rice

- 6 green onions, chopped

- ½ pound baby Bella mushrooms

- 2 cups of water

- 2 tablespoons olive oil

- 2 garlic cloves, minced

Directions:

1. In your slow cooker, mix the rice with garlic, onions, oil, mushrooms, water, toss, cover, and cook on Low for 3 hours. Stir the pilaf one more time, divide between plates and serve.

Nutrition:

Calories 151

Fat 5.1g

Sodium 9mg

Carbohydrate 23.3g

Fiber 2.6g

Sugars 1.7g

Protein 5.2g

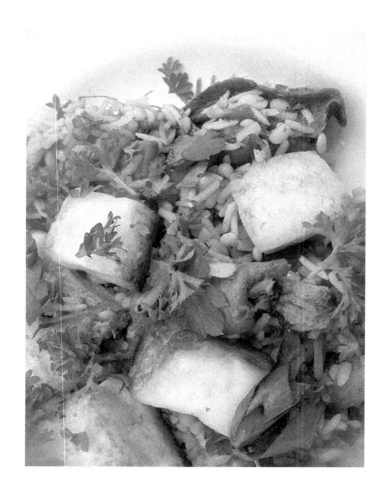

Parsley Fennel

Preparation time: 10 minutes

Cooking time: 2 hours and 30 minutes

Servings: 4

Ingredients:

- 2 fennel bulbs, sliced

- Juice and zest of 1 lime

- 2 teaspoons avocado oil

- ½ teaspoon turmeric powder

- 1 tablespoon parsley, chopped

- ¼ cup veggie stock, low-sodium

Directions:

1. In a slow cooker, combine the fennel with the lime juice, zest, and the other ingredients, cook on Low within 2 hours and 30 minutes. Serve.

Nutrition:

Calories 47

Fat 0.6g

Sodium 71mg

Carbohydrate 10.8g

Protein 1.7g

Sweet Butternut

Preparation time: 10 minutes

Cooking time: 4 hours

Servings: 8

Ingredients:

- 1 cup carrots, chopped

- 1 tablespoon olive oil

- 1 yellow onion, chopped

- ½ teaspoon stevia

- 1 garlic clove, minced

- ½ teaspoon curry powder

- 1 butternut squash, cubed

- 2 and ½ cups low-sodium veggie stock

- ½ cup basmati rice

- ¾ cup of coconut milk

- ½ teaspoon cinnamon powder

- ¼ teaspoon ginger, grated

Directions:

1. Heat-up, a pan with the oil over medium-high heat, add the oil, onion, garlic, stevia, carrots, curry

powder, cinnamon, ginger, stir, and cook 5 minutes and transfer to your slow cooker.

2. Add squash, stock, and coconut milk, stir, cover, and cook on Low for 4 hours. Divide the butternut mix between plates and serve as a side dish.

Nutrition:

Calories 134

Fat 7.2g

Sodium 59mg

Carbohydrate 16.5g

Fiber 1.7g

Sugars 2.7g

Protein 1.8g

Mushroom Sausages

Preparation time: 10 minutes

Cooking time: 2 hours

Servings: 12

Ingredients:

- 6 celery ribs, chopped

- 1 pound no-sugar, beef sausage, chopped

- 2 tablespoons olive oil

- ½ pound mushrooms, chopped

- ½ cup sunflower seeds, peeled

- 1 cup low-sodium veggie stock

- 1 cup cranberries, dried

- 2 yellow onions, chopped

- 2 garlic cloves, minced

- 1 tablespoon sage, dried

- 1 whole-wheat bread loaf, cubed

Directions:

1. Heat-up a pan with the oil over medium-high heat, add beef, stir and brown for a few minutes. Add mushrooms, onion, celery, garlic, and sage, stir,

cook for a few more minutes and transfer to your slow cooker.

2. Add stock, cranberries, sunflower seeds, and the bread cubes; cover and cook on High for 2 hours. Stir the whole mix, divide between plates and serve as a side dish.

Nutrition:

Calories 188

Fat 13.8g

Sodium 489mg

Carbohydrate 8.2g

Fiber 1.9g

Protein 7.6g

Parsley Red Potatoes

Preparation time: 10 minutes

Cooking time: 6 hours

Servings: 8

Ingredients:

- 16 baby red potatoes, halved

- 2 cups low-sodium chicken stock

- 1 carrot, sliced

- 1 celery rib, chopped

- ¼ cup yellow onion, chopped

- 1 tablespoon parsley, chopped

- 2 tablespoons olive oil

- A pinch of black pepper

- 1 garlic clove minced

Directions:

1. In your slow cooker, mix the potatoes with the carrot, celery, onion, stock, parsley, garlic, oil, and black pepper, toss, cover, and cook on Low for 6 hours. Serve.

Nutrition:

Calories 257

Fat 9.5g

Sodium 845mg

Carbohydrate 43.4g

Protein 4.4g

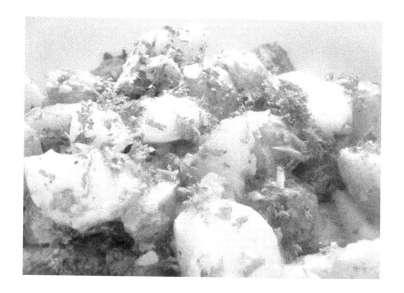

Jalapeno Black-Eyed Peas Mix

Preparation time: 10 minutes

Cooking time: 5 hours

Servings: 12

Ingredients:

- 17 ounces black-eyed peas

- 1 sweet red pepper, chopped

- ½ cup sausage, chopped

- 1 yellow onion, chopped

- 1 jalapeno, chopped

- 2 garlic cloves minced

- 6 cups of water

- ½ teaspoon cumin, ground

- A pinch of black pepper

- 2 tablespoons cilantro, chopped

Directions:

1. In your slow cooker, mix the peas with the sausage, onion, red pepper, jalapeno, garlic, cumin, black pepper, water, cilantro, cover, and cook low for 5 hours. Serve.

Nutrition:

Calories 75

Fat 3.5g

Sodium 94mg

Carbohydrate 7.2g

Fiber 1.7g

Sugars 0.9g

Protein 4.3g

Sour Cream Green Beans

Preparation time: 10 minutes

Cooking time: 4 hours

Servings: 8

Ingredients:

- 15 ounces green beans

- 14 ounces corn

- 4 ounces mushrooms, sliced

- 11 ounces cream of mushroom soup, low-fat and sodium-free

- ½ cup low-fat sour cream

- ½ cup almonds, chopped

- ½ cup low-fat cheddar cheese, shredded

Directions:

1. In your slow cooker, mix the green beans with the corn, mushrooms soup, mushrooms, almonds, cheese, sour cream, toss, cover, and cook on Low for 4 hours. Stir one more time, divide between plates and serve as a side dish.

Nutrition:

Calories360

Fat 12.7g

Sodium 220mg

Carbohydrate 58.3g

Fiber 10g

Sugars 10.3g

Protein 14g

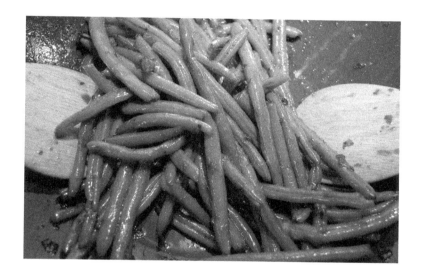

Cumin Brussels Sprouts

Preparation time: 10 minutes

Cooking time: 3 hours

Servings: 4

Ingredients:

- 1 cup low-sodium veggie stock

- 1-pound Brussels sprouts, trimmed and halved

- 1 teaspoon rosemary, dried

- 1 teaspoon cumin, ground

- 1 tablespoon mint, chopped

Directions:

1. In your slow cooker, combine the sprouts with the stock and the other ingredients, cook on Low within 3 hours. Serve.

Nutrition:

Calories 56

Fat 0.6g

Sodium 65mg

Carbohydrate 11.4g

Fiber 4.5g

Sugars 2.7g

Protein 4g

Peach and Carrots

Preparation time: 10 minutes

Cooking time: 6 hours

Servings: 6

Ingredients:

- 2 pounds small carrots, peeled

- ½ cup low-fat butter, melted

- ½ cup canned peach, unsweetened

- 2 tablespoons cornstarch

- 3 tablespoons stevia

- 2 tablespoons water

- ½ teaspoon cinnamon powder

- 1 teaspoon vanilla extract

- A pinch of nutmeg, ground

Directions:

1. In your slow cooker, mix the carrots with the butter, peach, stevia, cinnamon, vanilla, nutmeg, and cornstarch mixed with water, toss, cover, and cook on Low for 6 hours. Toss the carrots one more time, divide between plates and serve as a side dish.

Nutrition:

Calories139

Fat 10.7g

Sodium 199mg

Carbohydrate 35.4g

Fiber 4.2g

Sugars 6.9g

Protein 3.8g

Baby Spinach and Grains Mix

Preparation time: 10 minutes

Cooking time: 4 hours

Servings: 12

Ingredients:

- 1 butternut squash, peeled and cubed

- 1 cup whole-grain blend, uncooked

- 12 ounces low-sodium veggie stock

- 6 ounces baby spinach

- 1 yellow onion, chopped

- 3 garlic cloves, minced

- ½ cup of water

- 2 teaspoons thyme, chopped

- A pinch of black pepper

Directions:

1. In your slow cooker, mix the squash with whole grain, onion, garlic, water, thyme, black pepper, stock, spinach, cover, and cook on Low for 4 hours. Serve.

Nutrition:

Calories78

Fat 0.6g

Sodium 259mg

Carbohydrate 16.4g

Fiber 1.8g

Sugars 2g

Protein 2.5g

Quinoa Curry

Preparation time: 15 minutes

Cooking time: 4 hours

Servings: 8

Ingredients:

- 1 chopped Sweet Potato

- 2 cups Green Beans

- ½ diced onion (white)

- 1 diced Carrot

- 15 oz Chick Peas (organic and drained)

- 28 oz. Tomatoes (diced)

- 29 oz Coconut Milk

- 2 minced cloves of garlic

- ¼ cup Quinoa

- 1 tbs. Turmeric (ground)

- 1 tbsp. Ginger (grated)

- 1 ½ cups Water

- 1 tsp. of Chili Flakes

- 2 tsp. of Tamari Sauce

Directions:

1. Put all the listed fixing in the slow cooker. Add 1 cup of water. Stir well. Cook on "high" for 4 hrs. Serve with rice.

Nutrition:

Calories 297

Fat 18 g

Sodium 364 mg

Carbohydrates 9 mg

Protein 28 g